POSTPRANDIAL SOMNOLENCE:

The Science Behind After-Meal Sleepiness

Carlos k. Lewis

1

TABLE OF CONTENTS

Postprandial somnolence

CHAPTER 1: INTRODUCTION

Postprandial somnolence, also referred to as "food coma," is an interesting physiological phenomenon that appears as a feeling of fatigue or drowsiness after eating.

Researchers, nutritionists, and individuals have all become interested in this complex relationship between eating and fatigue, which has led to studies into its underlying mechanisms and possible health implications.

"Somnolence" is a state of sleepiness or drowsiness, whereas "postprandial" refers to the time after eating. Not only are reports of post-meal drowsiness anecdotal, but scientific research has been conducted to identify the complex network of factors causing this phenomenon.

As a result of increased blood flow to the digestive organs, the secretion of digestive enzymes, and the absorption of nutrients, the digestive process itself requires a substantial energy expenditure. This physiological activity may affect alertness and cognitive function by taking resources away from other bodily processes.

Furthermore, the meal's composition is a major factor in determining how much postprandial somnolence occurs. Post-meal fatigue has been associated with higher levels of glycemic index meals, which are high in carbohydrates. Lethargy may result from the fast rise and subsequent fall in blood sugar levels following such meals.

Meals with enough fats and protein, on the other hand, might have a more moderate effect on postprandial alertness.

Understanding postprandial somnolence extends beyond mere curiosity about why one might feel sluggish after a satisfying meal. Researchers explore its potential implications for various aspects of health, including its association with conditions such as insulin resistance and metabolic syndrome.

Furthermore, the impact of postprandial somnolence on cognitive function and productivity has garnered attention in fields ranging from nutrition science to workplace ergonomics.

In this exploration, we delve into the intricacies of postprandial somnolence, examining the physiological processes at play, the influence of dietary factors, and potential implications for health and daily functioning.

Through this comprehensive investigation, we aim to shed light on a phenomenon that resonates with virtually every individual and to provide insights into how we can better navigate the delicate balance between satisfying meals and sustaining energy levels throughout the day.

1.1 Definition

Postprandial somnolence, commonly known as food coma, refers to the state of drowsiness or lethargy that individuals may experience after consuming a meal, particularly a large or carbohydrate-rich one.

This phenomenon is attributed to the body's physiological response to the digestive process. After eating, blood is directed to the digestive system to facilitate nutrient absorption and processing, leading to a temporary decrease in blood flow to other organs, including the brain.

When digestion occurs, the parasympathetic nervous system becomes more active, encouraging relaxation and directing energy toward metabolic functions. Simultaneously, there is a rise in the synthesis and release of serotonin, which adds to a feeling of calm and possible sleepiness.

Furthermore, the release of insulin in response to elevated blood sugar levels can improve the brain's absorption of specific amino acids, like tryptophan. The hormones serotonin and melatonin, which are both linked to the control of sleep, are precursors to tryptophan.

Factors influencing the severity of postprandial somnolence include the composition and size of the meal, with larger, carbohydrate-dense meals more likely to induce pronounced drowsiness.

While postprandial somnolence is a normal physiological response, excessive or persistent fatigue after eating could be indicative of other underlying health issues and may warrant further investigation.

The process begins with the act of eating, triggering a cascade of physiological changes. As food is consumed, the digestive system mobilizes to break down complex nutrients into simpler forms for absorption.

To support this process, blood flow is redirected to the digestive organs, including the stomach and intestines. This diversion of blood flow away from other bodily functions, including the brain, contributes to a temporary decrease in alertness and an increase in feelings of tiredness.

The size and composition of the meal also play a role in the intensity of postprandial somnolence. Larger meals and those rich in carbohydrates are more likely to induce a more significant and prolonged feeling of drowsiness.

Carbohydrates, in particular, stimulate the release of insulin and promote the entry of tryptophan into the brain.

While postprandial somnolence is a normal and temporary experience for many people, individuals may vary in their susceptibility to this phenomenon.

Additionally, if excessive fatigue or persistent drowsiness after meals becomes a regular occurrence, it could be indicative of other health factors such as insulin resistance, sleep disorders, or digestive issues, warranting further attention and evaluation.

1.2 Occurrence and frequency

Occurrence:

1. Physiological Mechanisms: Postprandial somnolence occurs due to physiological changes during the digestion process. When you eat, blood flow is redirected to the digestive system, and the body expends energy on breaking down food. This redistribution of resources can lead to a temporary decrease in alertness.

2. Neurotransmitter Release: The consumption of food triggers the release of neurotransmitters like serotonin and melatonin. These chemicals are associated with relaxation and sleep. The increase in their levels contributes to the feeling of drowsiness after a meal.

3. Insulin and Tryptophan: Meals, especially those rich in carbohydrates, stimulate insulin release. Insulin promotes the uptake of amino acids into cells, increasing the availability of tryptophan. Tryptophan is a precursor to serotonin and melatonin, further enhancing the sleep-inducing effect.

4. Blood Sugar Fluctuations: Eating can cause a temporary spike in blood sugar levels, followed by a subsequent drop. This fluctuation may contribute to feelings of lethargy and drowsiness.

Frequency:

1. Individual Variations: The frequency of postprandial somnolence varies among individuals. Factors such as age, metabolism, and overall health influence how intensely someone experiences drowsiness after eating.

2. Meal Composition:The type of food consumed plays a crucial role. High-

carbohydrate and high-fat meals tend to induce more pronounced postprandial somnolence compared to balanced meals with protein, fiber, and moderate carbohydrate content.

3. Meal Size: Larger meals generally result in a more significant postprandial somnolence effect. The body expends more energy on digesting larger quantities of food, intensifying the temporary drowsiness.

4. Cultural Practices: Some cultures embrace post-meal rest or napping as a norm. These practices acknowledge and accommodate the natural inclination for drowsiness after eating.

5. Hydration and Lifestyle: Dehydration can exacerbate feelings of fatigue. Maintaining proper hydration and incorporating regular physical activity into one's lifestyle can influence the frequency and intensity of postprandial somnolence.

Postprandial somnolence

While postprandial somnolence is a normal part of the digestive process, persistent or extreme drowsiness after meals might warrant attention, as it could be indicative of underlying health issues such as insulin resistance or sleep disorders.

Adopting healthy eating habits and lifestyle choices can help manage and regulate the occurrence of postprandial somnolence.

CHAPTER 2: MECHANISMS OF POSTPRANDIAL SOMNOLENCE

Postprandial somnolence, or the feeling of drowsiness after eating, involves intricate physiological processes. Here's a more detailed exploration of the mechanisms:

1. Insulin and Amino Acids:After a meal, especially one rich in carbohydrates, the body releases insulin to facilitate the uptake of glucose into cells. Simultaneously, amino acids, including tryptophan, enter the brain. Tryptophan is a precursor to serotonin, a neurotransmitter that influences mood and sleep.

2. Serotonin and Melatonin Production: Increased tryptophan in the brain leads to higher serotonin levels. Serotonin can be converted into melatonin, a hormone that regulates sleep-wake

cycles. Elevated melatonin contributes to the feeling of drowsiness.

3. Neurotransmitter Balance: The interplay of neurotransmitters like serotonin, dopamine, and norepinephrine influences alertness and relaxation. The postprandial state alters this balance, favoring neurotransmitters associated with relaxation and sleep.

4. Parasympathetic Nervous System Activation: The parasympathetic nervous system, activated during digestion, promotes a "rest and digest" state. Increased activity in this system redirects blood flow to the digestive organs, potentially reducing blood flow to the brain and contributing to feelings of lethargy.

5. Hormonal Changes:Hormones like cholecystokinin (CCK) are released in response to food intake. CCK signals satiety and may contribute to the overall relaxation response associated with postprandial somnolence.

6. Blood Flow Redistribution: The demands of the digestive process require increased blood flow to the gastrointestinal system. This temporary shift in blood flow away from other areas of the body, including the brain and muscles, can contribute to a sense of fatigue.

7. Meal Composition and Size:The composition and size of the meal influence postprandial somnolence. Large meals, especially those high in fats and simple carbohydrates, may intensify feelings of tiredness due to the increased metabolic load on the digestive system.

8. Circadian Rhythms: The body's internal clock, or circadian rhythms, affects the timing of physiological processes. Eating during a circadian low, such as the afternoon for many individuals, can enhance the natural tendency to feel drowsy.

In essence, postprandial somnolence is a multifaceted phenomenon involving the intricate coordination of hormones, neurotransmitters, and physiological responses. The specific impact can vary based on individual factors, the type of meal consumed, and the time of day.

2.1 Digestive process

Several factors contribute to this phenomenon, including the digestive processes.

When you eat, your body directs more blood to the digestive system to aid in the breakdown of food. This increased blood flow can lead to a temporary decrease in blood flow to the brain, potentially causing feelings of lethargy. Additionally, the process of digestion requires energy, and the body redirects resources to support these metabolic activities.

The consumption of carbohydrates, especially in large quantities, can play a significant role in postprandial somnolence.

Carbohydrates stimulate the release of insulin, which promotes the uptake of certain amino acids into cells. This, in turn, facilitates the entry of tryptophan into the brain. Tryptophan is a precursor to serotonin and melatonin, neurotransmitters associated with relaxation and sleep.

Furthermore, meals rich in fats and proteins can also contribute to postprandial somnolence. These macronutrients trigger the release of various hormones and digestive enzymes, further intensifying the body's metabolic activities and potentially contributing to feelings of fatigue.

In summary, postprandial somnolence involves a complex interplay of factors, including increased blood flow to the digestive system, energy expenditure during digestion, and the impact of specific nutrients on neurotransmitter levels.

2.2 Hormonal influences

Hormonal influences on postprandial somnolence are notable, with several hormones playing key roles in regulating the body's response to food intake. Here are some of the primary hormones involved:

1. Insulin: After a meal, especially one rich in carbohydrates, the pancreas releases insulin to help cells absorb glucose for energy. The increased insulin levels can enhance the uptake of certain amino acids into cells, promoting the entry of tryptophan into the brain.

Tryptophan is a precursor to serotonin and melatonin, which have relaxing and sleep-inducing effects.

2. Melatonin: While melatonin is commonly associated with regulating the sleep-wake cycle, its levels can also be influenced by food intake. Certain foods contain melatonin or can stimulate its production. The increase in melatonin levels during digestion may contribute to feelings of drowsiness.

3. Serotonin: As mentioned earlier, tryptophan, an amino acid derived from food, is a precursor

to serotonin. Serotonin is a neurotransmitter that can have calming and mood-stabilizing effects. Elevated serotonin levels may contribute to the sense of relaxation and drowsiness after a meal.

4. Ghrelin:Often referred to as the hunger hormone, ghrelin levels typically rise before meals and decrease afterward. However, in some individuals, ghrelin levels may remain elevated postprandially, potentially contributing to feelings of drowsiness.

5. Cholecystokinin (CCK): Released in response to the presence of fats and proteins in the digestive system, CCK plays a role in regulating digestion by slowing down the emptying of the stomach. This delay in gastric emptying can contribute to a sense of fullness and, consequently, postprandial somnolence.

These hormonal responses, combined with other factors like increased blood flow to the digestive system and energy expenditure during digestion, collectively contribute to the phenomenon of postprandial somnolence. Individual variations in hormone sensitivity and meal composition can influence the degree to which these hormonal factors contribute to feelings of drowsiness after eating.

2.3 Neural pathways

The neural pathways involved in postprandial somnolence are complex and interconnected, involving various regions of the brain that regulate both the digestive process and sleep-wake cycles. Here's a simplified overview:

1. Brainstem Activation: The brainstem, particularly the medulla oblongata, plays a crucial role in regulating autonomic functions, including digestion and sleep. It receives signals from the gastrointestinal tract indicating the presence of food and initiates the release of digestive enzymes and hormones.

2. Vagus Nerve Stimulation: The vagus nerve, a major component of the parasympathetic nervous system, is essential in the regulation of digestion. It helps stimulate the release of digestive enzymes and promotes the absorption of nutrients. Activation of the vagus nerve is associated with a restful and relaxed state, contributing to the overall calming effect after a meal.

3. Hypothalamus Integration: The hypothalamus, a key regulatory center in the brain, integrates signals related to hunger, satiety, and sleep. It receives information from the digestive system, including hormonal signals such as insulin and ghrelin. The hypothalamus is also involved in the regulation of the sleep-wake cycle.

4. Serotonin and Melatonin Production: The gut produces a significant amount of serotonin, a neurotransmitter associated with mood and relaxation. Serotonin can be converted into melatonin, a hormone that regulates sleep. The increased availability of tryptophan, a precursor

to serotonin, after a meal contributes to the synthesis of these sleep-inducing compounds.

5. Circadian Rhythms: The body's internal clock, regulated by the suprachiasmatic nucleus in the hypothalamus, influences both the timing of meals and the sleep-wake cycle.

The circadian system can modulate the impact of postprandial changes on alertness and sleepiness, with certain times of the day being more conducive to postprandial somnolence.

6. Thalamus and Cortex Interaction:The thalamus, a relay center in the brain, processes sensory information. After a meal, increased blood flow to the digestive system may divert resources away from the brain temporarily.

This, combined with hormonal and neurotransmitter changes, may influence the thalamus and cortical activity, contributing to feelings of drowsiness.

In summary, the neural pathways of postprandial somnolence involve intricate communication between the digestive system and various brain regions, integrating signals related to food intake, hormonal responses, and the regulation of sleep-wake cycles. Individual variations in these neural pathways may contribute to differences in how people experience postprandial somnolence.

CHAPTER 3: FACTORS CONTRIBUTING TO POSTPRANDIAL SOMNOLENCE

Postprandial somnolence, or the tendency to feel sleepy after eating, is influenced by various factors. The digestive process itself requires energy and redirects blood flow, contributing to a potential decrease in alertness.

Additionally, the release of insulin following carbohydrate consumption can increase tryptophan uptake, leading to the production of serotonin and melatonin, neurotransmitters associated with relaxation and sleep.

Activation of the parasympathetic nervous system during and after meals promotes a "rest and digest" response, enhancing feelings of drowsiness.

Fluctuations in blood sugar levels, particularly after consuming large, carbohydrate-rich meals, can also impact energy levels. Furthermore, meal composition, dehydration, and circadian rhythms contribute to the complex interplay of factors influencing postprandial somnolence.

3.1 Meal Composition

Meal composition significantly contributes to postprandial somnolence, influencing the body's physiological and biochemical responses after eating. Here's an elaboration on how different aspects of meal composition contribute to this phenomenon:

1. Carbohydrates:
   - Meals high in carbohydrates, particularly those with a high glycemic index, cause a rapid increase in blood glucose levels. This prompts the pancreas to release insulin, facilitating the

uptake of glucose into cells. Simultaneously, insulin promotes the entry of tryptophan into the brain. Tryptophan is a precursor to serotonin and melatonin, neurotransmitters associated with relaxation and sleep. Therefore, carbohydrate-rich meals can contribute to feelings of drowsiness.

2. Proteins:

- Foods rich in proteins contain amino acids, including tryptophan. While tryptophan is present in small amounts, its concentration relative to other amino acids increases after a protein-rich meal. Tryptophan's conversion into serotonin and melatonin can enhance feelings of relaxation and contribute to postprandial somnolence.

3. Fats:

- High-fat meals can delay gastric emptying, slowing the absorption of nutrients. This delayed digestion process can lead to a prolonged feeling of fullness and a diversion of blood flow to the digestive system. As a result, less blood and energy are available for other bodily functions, potentially contributing to drowsiness.

4. Meal Size and Caloric Intake:

- Larger meals and higher caloric intake require increased blood flow to the digestive system for proper digestion and absorption. This redirection of blood away from other bodily functions, including alertness, may contribute to the post-meal slump.

5. Nutrient Interaction:

- The combination of macronutrients in a meal can influence postprandial somnolence. For example, consuming carbohydrates with proteins may enhance the transport of tryptophan into the brain, potentially amplifying its sleep-inducing effects.

6. Insulin Response:

- The release of insulin in response to elevated blood glucose levels not only aids in glucose uptake but also facilitates the entry of amino acids, including tryptophan, into cells. This insulin-mediated process contributes to the synthesis of serotonin and melatonin, reinforcing the sleep-promoting effects.

7. Hydration Status:
  - Dehydration can exacerbate the feelings of fatigue and contribute to postprandial somnolence. Adequate hydration supports optimal digestion and nutrient absorption, helping to maintain overall energy levels.

Understanding the intricate interplay of these factors within meal composition provides insights into how dietary choices can impact postprandial somnolence. By making informed decisions about the types and sizes of meals, individuals can potentially manage and mitigate the intensity of the post-meal drowsiness.

3.2 Portion size

Portion size plays a crucial role in contributing to postprandial somnolence, affecting various physiological processes associated with digestion and energy metabolism. Here's an elaboration on how portion size influences the post-meal drowsiness:

1. Increased Blood Flow to Digestive System:
   - Larger portion sizes require more extensive digestive efforts, prompting increased blood flow to the gastrointestinal system. This redistribution of blood can temporarily divert resources away from other bodily functions, including those related to alertness and wakefulness.

The heightened demand for blood in the digestive organs may contribute to feelings of lethargy.

2. Energy Expenditure:
   - Digesting a larger meal demands more energy from the body. As energy is directed toward breaking down and absorbing nutrients, there can be a corresponding decrease in available energy for other activities.

This can lead to a general sense of fatigue and drowsiness following a large meal.

3. Insulin Release:
   - Larger meals often result in a more significant spike in blood glucose levels, triggering a corresponding increase in insulin secretion. Insulin facilitates the uptake of glucose into cells, but it also promotes the entry of amino acids like tryptophan into the brain.

The subsequent increase in serotonin and melatonin synthesis can contribute to feelings of relaxation and drowsiness.

4. Gastric Distension:
   - A larger portion size can lead to increased gastric distension, stretching the stomach walls. This stretching activates receptors that signal to the brain that the stomach is full. The resulting sensation of fullness can contribute to the overall sense of lethargy and drowsiness.

5. Extended Digestive Process:

- Larger meals take longer to digest, leading to an extended period of increased metabolic activity in the digestive system. This prolonged digestion process may further contribute to a sustained decrease in energy levels and increased feelings of drowsiness.

6. Circadian Rhythms:
- The body's circadian rhythms, which influence sleep-wake cycles, can be influenced by meal timing and size. Consuming a large meal close to bedtime may disrupt the natural drop in core body temperature that occurs as part of the sleep-wake cycle, potentially leading to increased drowsiness.

7. Postprandial Hyperglycemia:
- Larger meals can contribute to postprandial hyperglycemia, where blood glucose levels remain elevated for an extended period after eating. This can lead to fluctuations in energy levels and contribute to feelings of fatigue and drowsiness.

In summary, portion size influences postprandial somnolence through its impact on blood flow, energy expenditure, hormonal responses, and the duration of the digestive process. By being mindful of portion sizes, individuals can potentially manage and mitigate the intensity of post-meal drowsiness, promoting better overall alertness and well-being.

3.3 Timing of meals

The timing of meals plays a significant role in contributing to postprandial somnolence, influencing the body's circadian rhythms, hormonal fluctuations, and overall energy levels. Here's an elaboration on how meal timing contributes to the phenomenon of feeling drowsy after eating:

1. Circadian Rhythms:
   - The body follows a natural circadian rhythm that regulates various physiological processes, including sleep-wake cycles. Eating meals at

irregular times or consuming a large meal close to bedtime can disrupt these circadian rhythms, potentially leading to increased feelings of drowsiness.

2. Sleep-Wake Cycle Disruption:

- Consuming a heavy meal late in the evening can interfere with the body's natural transition to sleep. The digestive process requires energy and may elevate core body temperature, both of which can counteract the body's preparation for sleep. This disruption to the sleep-wake cycle can contribute to postprandial somnolence.

3. Insulin Response and Blood Glucose Levels:

- The timing of meals influences the body's insulin response and blood glucose levels. Consuming a meal, especially one high in carbohydrates, can lead to an increase in blood glucose levels.

If this occurs too close to bedtime, it can trigger an insulin response that facilitates the entry of tryptophan into the brain, promoting the synthesis of serotonin and melatonin, contributing to feelings of relaxation and drowsiness.

4. Daytime Alertness:

- Consuming a large or rich meal during the daytime can also impact alertness. The body typically experiences a natural dip in energy levels in the early afternoon, often referred to as the post-lunch dip. Eating a heavy meal during this time may exacerbate feelings of drowsiness.

5. Meal Size and Composition:

- The combination of meal size and composition interacts with meal timing. For example, a large, high-carbohydrate meal close to bedtime can have a more pronounced impact on postprandial somnolence than a smaller, balanced meal consumed earlier in the day.

6. Gastric Emptying:

- The rate at which the stomach empties its contents into the small intestine can be influenced by meal timing. Eating too close to bedtime may result in slower gastric emptying, prolonging the digestive process and potentially contributing to feelings of fullness and drowsiness.

7. Hydration and Electrolyte Balance:
 - The timing of fluid intake with meals can impact hydration and electrolyte balance. Dehydration can exacerbate feelings of fatigue, so it's important to consider fluid intake in relation to meal timing.

In summary, the timing of meals can affect the body's natural rhythms, hormonal responses, and energy levels, all of which contribute to postprandial somnolence.

 Being mindful of meal timing and considering factors such as circadian rhythms and the body's natural sleep-wake cycles can help individuals manage and potentially reduce post-meal drowsiness.

Postprandial somnolence

CHAPTER 4: IMPACT ON DAILY LIFE

The impact of postprandial somnolence on daily life can vary:

1. Productivity Dips:After consuming a heavy meal, individuals may experience a decline in alertness and concentration. This can affect work or daily tasks, leading to reduced productivity.

2. Impaired Performance:Activities requiring mental acuity or quick reflexes may be compromised during postprandial somnolence. Driving or operating heavy machinery immediately after a meal might pose risks.

3. Mood Changes: The sluggish feeling post-meal can influence mood, potentially leading to irritability or a lack of motivation to engage in activities.

4. Energy Drain: Instead of feeling recharged after a meal, some individuals may find themselves feeling more tired, impacting their ability to engage in physical activities or exercise.

5. Sleep Disruption at Night:Experiencing postprandial somnolence too close to bedtime can disrupt nighttime sleep patterns, potentially leading to insomnia or restless sleep.

6. Weight Management Challenges:Regular occurrences of postprandial somnolence may contribute to weight gain if individuals are less inclined to engage in physical activity after meals.

7. Cultural and Social Factors: In some cultures, it is customary to take short naps, known as siestas, after midday meals. This practice may align with postprandial somnolence and can be considered a cultural adaptation to the body's natural post-meal response.

It's important to note that the severity of postprandial somnolence varies among individuals and is influenced by factors such as meal composition, portion size, and overall health. Strategies like consuming smaller, balanced meals and staying hydrated can help mitigate its impact on daily life.

4.1 work and productivity

Postprandial somnolence, commonly known as the feeling of drowsiness or fatigue after a meal, can impact work and productivity in various ways. The physiological response to eating, particularly larger meals, involves increased blood flow to the digestive system, leading to a temporary decrease in blood flow to the brain. This shift can result in a feeling of lethargy and reduced alertness.

In a work setting, experiencing postprandial somnolence can lead to decreased concentration, impaired cognitive function, and a general decline in productivity. Employees may find it challenging to focus on tasks, make decisions, or maintain the same level of efficiency after a meal, especially during the post-lunch period when this phenomenon is commonly observed.

Employers may need to consider factors such as the timing and content of meals provided in the workplace to optimize employee alertness and productivity. Encouraging light, balanced meals and providing spaces for short breaks or even a brief walk after meals can help mitigate the impact of postprandial somnolence on work performance.

Additionally, individuals can adopt personal strategies, such as choosing nutritious snacks and staying hydrated, to manage the effects of post-meal fatigue in their daily work routines.

4.2 lifestyle considerations

Postprandial somnolence, or the drowsiness experienced after a meal, can be influenced by various lifestyle considerations, impacting our daily lives in several ways:

1. Meal Composition and Size:The type and size of the meal can contribute to postprandial somnolence. Heavier, carbohydrate-rich meals may induce a more pronounced drowsiness. Therefore, choosing lighter, balanced meals with a mix of proteins, fats, and carbohydrates can help mitigate this effect.

2. Meal Timing: The timing of meals can influence the degree of postprandial somnolence. Consuming a large meal during work hours, especially in the afternoon, might affect productivity due to the associated drowsiness. Strategic meal planning, such as having smaller, nutrient-dense snacks, may help manage energy levels more effectively.

3. Hydration:Dehydration can exacerbate feelings of fatigue. Maintaining adequate hydration throughout the day is essential for overall well-being and can help reduce the impact of postprandial somnolence.

4. Physical Activity:Engaging in light physical activity after a meal, such as taking a short walk, can promote digestion and alleviate the drowsiness associated with postprandial somnolence. Incorporating regular exercise into your daily routine can also contribute to increased overall alertness.

5. Sleep Quality: The overall quality of sleep the night before can influence postprandial somnolence. Individuals who experience insufficient or poor-quality sleep may be more prone to feeling excessively tired after meals.

6. Stress Levels: High stress levels can amplify the effects of postprandial somnolence. Managing stress through relaxation techniques,

mindfulness, or brief breaks during the day can positively impact energy levels.

7. Caffeine and Stimulant Intake:The consumption of caffeinated beverages or other stimulants can either alleviate or exacerbate postprandial somnolence, depending on individual tolerance levels and timing. Moderation and awareness of how these substances affect your body can be key.

8. Work Environment:The nature of your work environment can influence how you manage postprandial somnolence. Jobs that allow for flexible schedules or provide spaces for short breaks may accommodate the need to cope with drowsiness more effectively.

By considering these lifestyle factors, individuals can make informed choices to minimize the impact of postprandial somnolence on their daily activities and overall productivity.

CHAPTER 5: MANAGING POSTPRANDIAL SOMNOLENCE

Managing postprandial somnolence, or food-induced drowsiness, involves adopting lifestyle and dietary practices to minimize its impact. Here's a detailed guide:

1. Meal Composition:
   - Balanced Nutrients:Include a mix of carbohydrates, proteins, and healthy fats in your meals. This balance helps regulate blood sugar levels, preventing sharp spikes and crashes.
   - **Fiber-rich Foods:** Choose whole grains, fruits, and vegetables for sustained energy release.

2. Portion Control:
   - **Moderate Portions:** Avoid overeating by controlling portion sizes. Large meals can lead

to a more significant release of insulin, contributing to drowsiness.

3. Hydration:
   - *Pre and Post-Meal Hydration:Drink water before and after meals. Adequate hydration supports digestion and helps prevent dehydration-related fatigue.

4. Meal Timing:
   - Strategic Scheduling:Plan meals around activities that require alertness. Avoid heavy meals close to tasks demanding focus, such as work or driving.

5. Nutrient-Rich Foods:
   - Choose Wisely:Prioritize nutrient-dense foods over processed or sugary options. These provide sustained energy without the energy crashes associated with refined sugars.

6. Physical Activity:
   - Post-Meal Walks: Engage in light physical activity after meals, like a short walk. This aids

digestion and can mitigate postprandial drowsiness.

7. Caffeine Moderation:
   - Mindful Consumption: Limit caffeine intake, especially in the afternoon. While caffeine can provide a temporary energy boost, excessive consumption or late ingestion may interfere with sleep.

8. Mindful Eating:
   - Slow and Enjoyable: Eat slowly, savoring each bite. This allows your body to better manage the digestive process and can reduce the likelihood of feeling excessively sleepy after eating.

9. Napping:
   - Short Naps:If possible, consider a short nap (15-20 minutes) after a meal. Longer naps can interfere with nighttime sleep patterns.

10. Consistent Sleep Schedule:

- prioritize Sleep: Ensure you get sufficient and quality nighttime sleep. Establish and maintain a consistent sleep routine to support overall alertness during the day.

11. Observation and Adjustments:
- self-awareness:Pay attention to how your body responds to different foods and meal patterns. Adjust your diet and lifestyle based on your individual needs and responses.

12. Professional Consultation:
- Persistent Issues:If postprandial somnolence persists despite lifestyle changes, consult with a healthcare professional. It could be indicative of underlying health issues that require attention.

By incorporating these practices into your daily routine, you can better manage postprandial somnolence and promote sustained energy levels throughout the day.

5.1 Dietary Modifications

Certainly! Postprandial somnolence, commonly known as food-induced drowsiness or the "after-meal slump," is a natural physiological response to eating. However, certain dietary modifications can help manage and alleviate this condition:

1. Balanced Meals: Opt for well-balanced meals that include a mix of carbohydrates, proteins, and fats. This combination helps regulate blood sugar levels and prevents rapid spikes and crashes, reducing the likelihood of post-meal drowsiness.

2. Complex Carbohydrates:Choose complex carbohydrates with a low glycemic index (GI), such as whole grains, legumes, and vegetables. These foods release glucose gradually, providing a steady supply of energy and preventing sudden blood sugar fluctuations.

3. Protein-Rich Foods: Incorporate protein-rich foods like lean meats, fish, eggs, dairy, and

plant-based proteins into your meals. Protein helps slow down the digestion of carbohydrates, promoting a more gradual release of energy.

4. Fiber Intake:Include high-fiber foods in your diet, such as fruits, vegetables, and whole grains. Fiber not only contributes to overall digestive health but also helps stabilize blood sugar levels and maintain energy levels.

5. Hydration:Stay well-hydrated throughout the day. Dehydration can contribute to feelings of fatigue. Water helps in the digestion process and supports overall bodily functions, potentially reducing postprandial somnolence.

6. Moderate Portion Sizes:Overeating can lead to increased blood flow to the digestive system, diverting blood away from other parts of the body and causing drowsiness. Aim for moderate portion sizes to avoid overwhelming your digestive system.

7. Mindful Eating:Practice mindful eating by savoring each bite, chewing thoroughly, and paying attention to hunger and fullness cues. This can enhance the digestive process and promote a more balanced release of energy.

8. Limit Sugary Foods and Drinks: Minimize the intake of sugary foods and beverages, as they can cause rapid spikes and subsequent crashes in blood sugar levels, contributing to postprandial somnolence.

9. Caffeine Consideration:While some people find that a moderate amount of caffeine can help counteract drowsiness, it's essential to be mindful of individual tolerance and not consume excessive amounts, especially later in the day.

Remember that individual responses to food can vary, so it may be helpful to experiment with these dietary modifications to find the combination that works best for you. If persistent or severe, it's advisable to consult with a healthcare professional for personalized advice.

5.2 Physical Activity

Certainly! Physical activity can be an effective strategy in managing postprandial somnolence, the drowsiness or fatigue experienced after meals. Here's a detailed overview of how exercise can help:

1. Improved Blood Circulation: Engaging in physical activity, even a brisk walk, enhances blood circulation throughout the body. This increased blood flow can counteract the tendency for blood to pool in the digestive system after a meal, reducing feelings of sluggishness.

2. Enhanced Insulin Sensitivity:Regular physical activity improves insulin sensitivity, allowing cells to more efficiently take up glucose from the bloodstream. This can help stabilize blood sugar

levels and prevent the rapid spikes and crashes that contribute to post-meal drowsiness.

3. Stimulation of Brain Activity:Exercise triggers the release of neurotransmitters, such as dopamine and norepinephrine, which are associated with increased alertness and improved mood. This can counteract the lethargy often experienced after eating.

4. Promotion of Digestive Processes:Moderate physical activity can promote digestion by aiding the movement of food through the digestive tract. This may reduce the feeling of fullness and discomfort that can contribute to postprandial somnolence.

5. Energy Expenditure: Physical activity burns calories and increases overall energy expenditure. This can help prevent an excessive influx of energy from a large meal, potentially reducing the likelihood of feeling overly tired.

6. Timing of Exercise:While regular physical activity is beneficial, timing matters when it comes to managing postprandial somnolence. Avoid intense exercise immediately after eating, as it may divert blood flow away from the digestive system and lead to discomfort. Instead, consider a light walk or gentle stretching after meals.

7. Consistent Routine: Establishing a consistent exercise routine, including both aerobic and resistance training, can contribute to overall energy levels and help regulate bodily functions. Consistency is key in reaping the long-term benefits of physical activity.

8. Mind-Body Connection: Activities such as yoga and tai chi not only involve physical movement but also focus on breath control and mindfulness. These practices can promote relaxation and help alleviate stress, which may contribute to postprandial somnolence.

9. Hydration:Staying hydrated is crucial for overall energy levels and exercise performance. Water supports the digestive process and helps maintain optimal bodily functions, potentially reducing feelings of fatigue after meals.

10. Individual Preferences:The type and intensity of exercise that work best in managing postprandial somnolence can vary among individuals. It's important to choose activities that align with personal preferences and physical capabilities.

Incorporating regular physical activity into your routine, particularly after meals, can be a proactive and natural way to manage postprandial somnolence. As always, individuals with specific health concerns should consult with a healthcare professional before making significant changes to their exercise regimen.

5.3 Sleep Hygiene

Certainly! Sleep hygiene involves adopting practices and habits that promote quality and restful sleep. While it might seem unrelated, good sleep hygiene can actually contribute to managing postprandial somnolence. Here's how:

1. Consistent Sleep Schedule:Going to bed and waking up at the same time every day helps regulate the body's internal clock. Consistency in sleep patterns can improve overall sleep quality, making it less likely to experience excessive daytime sleepiness, including postprandial somnolence.

2. Adequate Nighttime Sleep:Ensure you get enough sleep at night. Adults typically need 7-9 hours of sleep for optimal functioning. Having a sufficient amount of nighttime sleep can reduce the propensity for daytime drowsiness, including after meals.

3. Avoiding Stimulants Before Bed: Limit the intake of stimulants, such as caffeine and

nicotine, particularly in the evening. These substances can interfere with the ability to fall asleep and may exacerbate postprandial somnolence.

4. Create a Relaxing Bedtime Routine:Establish a calming pre-sleep routine to signal to your body that it's time to wind down. This can include activities like reading, gentle stretching, or practicing relaxation techniques, helping reduce stress and promoting better sleep.

5. Optimal Sleep Environment: Ensure your sleep environment is conducive to rest. This includes a comfortable mattress and pillows, as well as a cool, dark, and quiet room.

Creating an ideal sleep environment can enhance the quality of your sleep and reduce daytime sleepiness.

6. Limit Naps: While short power naps can be beneficial, especially if you didn't get enough sleep at night, long or irregular napping during

the day can disrupt nighttime sleep patterns. If you experience postprandial somnolence, try to limit naps or keep them short.

7. Physical Activity:Regular exercise can contribute to better sleep quality. However, avoid vigorous exercise close to bedtime, as it may energize you rather than promote relaxation.

8. Healthy Eating Habits:Maintain a balanced and nutritious diet. Avoid heavy meals close to bedtime, as they may cause discomfort and disrupt sleep. Additionally, a well-nourished body is better equipped to regulate energy levels throughout the day.

9. Limit Screen Time Before Bed:Exposure to the blue light emitted by screens (phones, tablets, computers) can interfere with the production of the sleep hormone melatonin. Try to limit screen time at least an hour before bedtime.

10. Manage Stress: High stress levels can contribute to both sleep disturbances and postprandial somnolence. Incorporate stress-reducing activities into your daily routine, such as meditation, deep breathing, or mindfulness practices.

By prioritizing good sleep hygiene practices, you can enhance the overall quality of your sleep and potentially reduce the likelihood of experiencing postprandial somnolence.

If sleep-related issues persist, it's advisable to consult with a healthcare professional for personalized guidance and assessment.

CHAPTER 6: CLINICAL PERSPECTIVE

From a clinical perspective, postprandial somnolence, or food-induced drowsiness, involves a complex interplay of physiological, neurological, and psychological factors. Let's delve deeper into some key aspects:

1. Insulin and Glucose Dynamics:
   - Insulin Release:After a meal, there is a surge in insulin production to facilitate the uptake of glucose into cells. This can lead to a temporary drop in blood sugar levels, contributing to feelings of fatigue.

2. Neurotransmitters and Hormones:
   - Serotonin and Melatonin: Tryptophan, an amino acid found in many protein-containing foods, can increase serotonin levels. Serotonin, in turn, can be converted to melatonin, a

hormone associated with sleep regulation, potentially inducing drowsiness.

- **Cholecystokinin (CCK):** Released during digestion, CCK influences feelings of fullness and may contribute to postprandial somnolence.

3. Meal Composition:
- Carbohydrates:High-carbohydrate meals can stimulate the release of insulin and increase serotonin levels, affecting mood and promoting relaxation.
- **Fats:** Meals high in fats may delay gastric emptying, extending the digestive process and contributing to a sense of lethargy.

4. Blood Flow Redistribution:
- Gastrointestinal Blood Flow: After eating, blood is redirected to the digestive system to aid in nutrient absorption. This shift in blood flow may temporarily reduce blood supply to the brain, contributing to drowsiness.

5. Individual Variability:

- Metabolic Rate:Variations in metabolic rates among individuals can influence how quickly nutrients are processed, impacting the severity of postprandial somnolence.
- Circadian Rhythms:The body's natural circadian rhythm plays a role, with a natural dip in alertness often occurring in the early afternoon.

6. Medical Conditions:
- Insulin Resistance: Conditions such as insulin resistance can lead to fluctuations in blood sugar levels, potentially exacerbating postprandial somnolence.
- Gastrointestinal Disorders:Conditions affecting digestion, like irritable bowel syndrome (IBS), can impact nutrient absorption and contribute to fatigue.

7. Psychological Factors:
- Stress and Anxiety: Psychological factors, such as stress or anxiety, can modulate the impact of postprandial somnolence. Individuals

experiencing stress may be more prone to feelings of fatigue after eating.

Understanding these clinical perspectives is crucial for healthcare professionals when evaluating patients who report excessive postprandial somnolence.

Tailoring interventions based on individual health profiles, addressing dietary habits, and considering psychological factors can contribute to more effective management of this phenomenon.

6.1 Relationship to Medical Conditions

The relationship between postprandial somnolence (PPS) and various medical conditions underscores the complex interplay between physiological processes and health. Here's a detailed exploration:

1. Insulin Resistance and Diabetes:

- Connection: Individuals with insulin resistance or diabetes may experience fluctuations in blood sugar levels after meals. This can lead to an imbalance in insulin production, contributing to postprandial fatigue.

- Management: Managing blood sugar levels through dietary modifications, consistent insulin use (for diabetes), and regular physical activity is crucial.

2. Gastrointestinal Disorders:

- Influence on Digestion:Conditions like irritable bowel syndrome (IBS) or inflammatory bowel disease (IBD) can affect the digestive process, potentially leading to prolonged absorption of nutrients and an increased likelihood of postprandial somnolence.

- Management:Addressing the underlying gastrointestinal condition, adopting a suitable diet, and managing symptoms can mitigate the impact on postprandial well-being.

3. Sleep Disorders:

- Bidirectional Relationship:Certain sleep disorders, such as sleep apnea or insomnia, can influence postprandial somnolence. Disrupted sleep patterns may exacerbate the drowsiness experienced after meals.

- Management: Treating the underlying sleep disorder through lifestyle changes, behavioral interventions, or medical treatments can positively impact postprandial somnolence.

4. Nutritional Deficiencies:

- Impact on Energy Levels:Deficiencies in essential nutrients, such as iron or B-vitamins, can affect energy metabolism and contribute to overall fatigue, potentially intensifying postprandial somnolence.

- Management:Nutritional supplementation or dietary adjustments to address deficiencies can be part of the management strategy.

5. Chronic Fatigue Syndrome (CFS):

- Enhanced Sensitivity: Individuals with chronic fatigue syndrome may be more sensitive to fluctuations in energy levels, and postprandial somnolence can be more pronounced.

- Management:Managing CFS involves a multidisciplinary approach, addressing both physical and psychological aspects of fatigue.

6. Psychiatric Conditions:

- Depression and Anxiety:Mental health conditions, especially depression and anxiety, can influence energy levels and contribute to postprandial somnolence.

- **Management:** A combination of psychotherapy, medication, and lifestyle modifications may be employed to manage psychiatric conditions and their impact on postprandial well-being.

7. Medication Effects:

- sedating Medications:Certain medications, such as antihistamines or muscle relaxants, may have sedative effects and can contribute to increased postprandial somnolence.

- Management:Adjusting medication timing or exploring alternative medications with fewer sedative side effects can be considered.

Understanding the relationship between postprandial somnolence and various medical conditions is crucial for healthcare professionals in tailoring interventions.

A comprehensive approach that addresses both the underlying health condition and lifestyle factors can contribute to effective management and improved quality of life for individuals experiencing postprandial somnolence in the context of medical conditions.

6.2 Treatment options

The treatment of postprandial somnolence (PPS) often involves a combination of lifestyle modifications, dietary changes, and, in some cases, addressing underlying health conditions. Here's a detailed overview of treatment options:

1. Dietary Modifications:

- Balanced Meals: Encourage patients to consume well-balanced meals that include a combination of carbohydrates, proteins, and healthy fats. This can help stabilize blood sugar levels and reduce the likelihood of postprandial fatigue.

- Moderate Portions: Large meals can exacerbate postprandial somnolence. Advising patients to consume moderate-sized portions may help in managing this phenomenon.

2. Meal Timing:

- Consistent Schedule:Establishing a regular eating schedule can help regulate blood sugar levels and reduce the severity of postprandial somnolence.

- Avoiding Heavy Meals Before Tasks: If possible, patients may be advised to avoid heavy meals before engaging in activities that require high levels of alertness.

3. Nutrient Composition:

- Protein and Fiber:Encourage the consumption of protein-rich foods and dietary fiber. These components can promote a more gradual release of energy, minimizing rapid fluctuations in blood sugar levels.

4. Hydration:
   - Adequate Fluid Intake:Dehydration can contribute to feelings of fatigue. Ensuring patients maintain adequate fluid intake throughout the day can be beneficial.

5. Physical Activity:
   - Regular Exercise:Physical activity can enhance overall energy levels and help regulate blood sugar. Advising patients to engage in regular exercise, even a short walk after meals, can be beneficial.

6. Sleep Hygiene:
   - Consistent Sleep Schedule:Encourage patients to maintain a consistent sleep schedule, ensuring they get adequate and quality sleep at

night. Addressing any underlying sleep disorders is crucial.

7. Medical Management:
   - Blood Sugar Monitoring:For individuals with diabetes or insulin resistance, regular monitoring of blood sugar levels and adjustments to medication may be necessary.
   - **Medication Review:** If postprandial somnolence is exacerbated by sedating medications, a review of medications with the healthcare provider may be considered.

8. Addressing Underlying Health Conditions:
   - Treatment of Gastrointestinal Disorders:If gastrointestinal conditions contribute to PPS, managing and treating these conditions can be essential.
   - Management of Sleep Disorders:For individuals with sleep disorders, such as sleep apnea or insomnia, specific treatments targeted at improving sleep quality may be recommended.

9. Caffeine Intake:

- Moderate Consumption:While excessive caffeine intake can disrupt sleep patterns, moderate consumption may help alleviate postprandial drowsiness for some individuals.

10. Stress Management:

- Stress Reduction Techniques:Stress and anxiety can contribute to postprandial somnolence. Techniques such as mindfulness, meditation, or relaxation exercises may be beneficial.

Individual responses to these treatment options can vary, and a personalized approach, considering the patient's overall health, lifestyle, and specific contributing factors, is crucial. Collaborative decision-making with healthcare providers ensures a comprehensive and effective treatment plan for managing postprandial somnolence.

CHAPTER 7: FUTURE RESEARCH AND DEVELOPMENTS

While I don't have real-time updates, as of my last knowledge update in January 2022, postprandial somnolence, or the feeling of drowsiness after eating, has been a subject of ongoing research.

Scientists are exploring various aspects of this phenomenon, including its physiological mechanisms, impact on cognitive function, and potential interventions.

1. Physiological Mechanisms:
   - Researchers are investigating the intricate processes within the body that lead to postprandial somnolence. This includes studying changes in blood flow, hormonal responses

(such as insulin and melatonin), and neurotransmitter activity.

2. Neurotransmitter Involvement:
  - The role of neurotransmitters, particularly serotonin and tryptophan, is a focal point. Understanding how these chemicals influence brain function post-meal could provide insights into managing or preventing postprandial somnolence.

3. Impact on Cognitive Function:
  - Future studies may delve into the cognitive consequences of postprandial somnolence. Exploring how it affects alertness, attention, and overall cognitive performance could have implications for various aspects of daily life, including productivity and safety.

4. Individual Variability:
  - Recognizing that individuals vary in their susceptibility to postprandial somnolence, researchers may aim to identify genetic, lifestyle, and dietary factors that contribute to

this variability. This personalized approach could lead to targeted interventions.

5. Interventions and Management:
-   Developing strategies to mitigate postprandial somnolence is an active area of interest. This may involve dietary modifications, such as adjusting meal composition or timing, as well as exploring the potential of certain nutrients or supplements.

6. Clinical Relevance:
-   Understanding whether postprandial somnolence is a normal physiological response or if it has clinical implications is another avenue of exploration. This could involve investigating its association with conditions like diabetes, obesity, or sleep disorders.

7. Technology and Monitoring:
- Advancements in wearable technology and continuous monitoring tools may enable more comprehensive tracking of postprandial somnolence in real-world settings. This data

could provide a richer understanding of its patterns and triggers.

8. Behavioral Strategies:
-    Behavioral interventions, such as incorporating short physical activity breaks after meals or optimizing sleep hygiene, might be explored as practical approaches to counteracting postprandial somnolence.

In the coming years, interdisciplinary research involving nutrition, neuroscience, and medicine is likely to contribute to a more nuanced understanding of postprandial somnolence, potentially leading to innovative interventions and personalized recommendations.

 Always check the latest literature and scientific journals for the most recent developments in this field

www.ingramcontent.com/pod-product-compliance
Lightning Source LLC
Chambersburg PA
CBHW062244290526
45794CB00006B/2393